THE CURLY NATURAL HAIR FOR BEGINNERS

Step by Step Guide On Everything You Need To Know on How to Reverse Damage Hair, Promote Hair Growth, and Achieve a Shinier Curly hair

Shannon Whitehead

TABLE OF CONTENT

CHAPTER 1: 4

WHAT TO KNOW ABOUT HAIR GROWTH 4

CHAPTER 2: 21

UNIQUE INGREDIENTS THAT WORKS EFFECTIVELY ON HAIR MASK.........21

CHAPTER 3: 26

RECIPES FOR HAIR MASK 26

CHAPTER 4: 31

WAYS YOU SHOULD APPLY HAIR MASK 31

CHAPTER 5: 36

THE KIND OF NATURAL SHAMPOO RECIPE YOU SHOULD AVOID 36

CHAPTER 6: 51

THE AFTER EFFECT OF USING APPLE CIDER VINEGAR FOR HAIR GROWTH 51

THE END.............................56

Chapter 1:

What to know about Hair growth

Do a Scalp massage to Stimulate boom

We spend lots of time and money piling on the products that it's clean to overlook in which hair growth starts off advanced: specifically, your scalp. "Much like authentic notable soil is critical to developing healthy flowers and flora, a wholesome scalp is a muse for wholesome hair growth. An easy way to stimulate hair growth at domestic is to provide you a scalp massage. This will grow blood go with the flow in your scalp, enhance the energy of your roots, and help nutrients get on your follicle quicker. You may provide yourself a scalp rubs down with dry hair, however, consisting of nutrient-rich oil to the mix will only double the blessings. (Just keep it to once in keeping with the week when you have oily roots).

Attempt an Egg Yolk mask to save you Breakage

Bauman notes that on average, hair grows about 1 / 4 to a half of an inch in keeping with month, and whilst we're able to boost up this method, we can have an effect on the quality of the hair shafts every follicle can produce (assume: thicker, stronger, shinier locks). There are things we can do to "stimulate a higher percentage of hair follicles inside the scalp, to be able to hold greater hair within the developing phase and make your head of hair thicker, healthier and fuller." Unsurprisingly, this makes the way you deal with your hair crucial to the natural hair increase. In case your hair breaks in advance then it gets past your shoulders, egg masks may be your savior. Eggs incorporate lecithin and protein, which give a boost to, nourish, and heal your strands.2plus; their excessive sulfur content might also even assist with dandruff.

To make the masks, mix eggs with tablespoons of olive oil. Add half a cup of water to dilute the aggregate (and make it a whole lot much less sticky). Follow the mask right now to dry, brushed hair, and depart it on for up to 1/2-hour. Then, shampoo and situation as everyday

Rinse with Cool Water to strengthen Hair

Similar to heat water can cause dryness on your pores and pores and skin; it can be adverse on your mane, too. Rinsing with cool water will assist in near up the cuticle and enhance hair follicles pre-styling. Cool water is terrific if you could manage it, but lukewarm is the subsequent fine factor in case you can't.

Do a heat Castor Oil treatment to promote boom

Castor oil is the unsung hero of the hair worldwide—you could also be tempted to ditch your coconut oil for it after analyzing this. To begin with, castor oil has anti-fungal and antibacterial houses to help fight scalp infections that prevent your hair from growing. Thirdly, it makes for a notable heat oil treatment—massaging the oil into your roots will help your scalp to drink up all of the nutrients and help promote hair boom.

To offer yourself a heat oil remedy, rub down the oil into your scalp after which apply it all the approaches to the ends of your strands

 Pile your hair at the pinnacle of your head, cowl it with a bathing cap, and blast your strands with a blow-dryer for 15 minutes. Enjoy unfastened to leap inside the shower and shampoo and circumstance as normal. You'll observe softer strands instantly.

Trade Hair boom supplements for healthful fats

 Sure, you could effortlessly pop a hair growth complement, but definitely, the phrases despite the fact that out on whether or not or now not or not they're an effective manner to help your hair increase quicker. Plus, they may be able to encompass pointless massive quantities of minerals and nutrients (ahem, biotin), that can sincerely wreak havoc in other ways (ahem, breakouts). For this purpose, eating your manner to longer hair is absolutely a higher, nutritionist-authorized manner to make your hair expand faster. Vitamins and minerals going on evidently in substances are less complicated in your body to utilize, and they may virtually deliver a healthier ratio of

Vitamins—simply the way Mother Nature meant.

In line with Pritchard, getting lots of healthful fats like omega-3s can bounce-begin hair increase.6 "healthy fats are essential to hair fitness when you consider that our bodies can't produce omega-three fatty acids on their personal. Consequently, it's vital to get that fat through our eating regimen. "They nourish hair follicles to present strands that sturdy, vibrant, lustrous glow."

Avoid Over-Shampooing to allow Your Hair repair

Relying on your hair type, the wide style of instances to shampoo your hair according to week will range. Thicker, coarser hair sorts can break out without washing their hair for some days at the identical time as thinner hair types also can find out their hair feels greasy even after at some point. In such instances, dry shampoo can paint wonders in absorbing extra grease as you look ahead to long strands.

DIY a Cinnamon-based mask to stimulate movement

Seems cinnamon is not the only accurate for sprinkling over your morning oatmeal. Thanks to its anti-microbial residences, it poses hair blessings too, inside the form of stimulating blood drift and nourishing strands. Combo the same additives cinnamon and coconut oil and comply with your hair, focusing on the roots. Permit it to do its factor for 45 minutes in advance than rinsing.

Trim Your Split Ends frequently

It might sound counterproductive in case you want your hair to develop longer, but ordinary trims get rid of dry, damaged break-up ends and are necessary for herbal, healthful growth. If left untreated, split ends can paintings their way up the shaft of your hair strand and motive even greater breakage, which means that the simplest factor growing maybe your frustration? in case your stylist takes to the air too much duration on every occasion you move in for a visit, your hair might not get longer, so be clear about your hair desires even as speaking with them. Relying on the state of affairs of your hair, your hairstyle, and your day-by-day recurring, you could want a trim anywhere from six weeks to six months. That stated, the better you cope with your hair on an everyday basis, the much less frequently you may want trims, and the longer your hair can develop naturally.

Brush gently when detangling

Not anything will check you're staying electricity like well detangling the knots for your hair; but, it is a critical step in growing your strands faster and one that truly shouldn't be rushed. If you have a bent too fast and haphazardly rip a brush through your hair and call it quits, you would probably want to rethink. Now not taking the right care whilst brushing can purpose your strands to interrupt off and cut up—quite lots the alternative of hair growth. With regards to brushing your hair, suppose: gradual and mild.

And, seems the brush you pick out makes a distinction. at the same time as a brush with steel, bristles have their purpose, a huge-tooth comb, a detangling brush, or a paddle brush with rounded bristles are all better options for lightly combing through knots and inflicting minimal breakage. Nearly as essential as what you use to comb your hair is whilst you select out to acquire this. In the desire to detangling after the shower (at the same time as the hair is most prone and fragile), comb thru your knots in advance before you wash your hair

Sleep on a Silk Pillowcase to keep away from Tangles

A silk or satin hair cover or pillowcase is better for the health of your hair as opposed to cotton if you need to take in all of the moisture out of your strands and cause tangles and breakage. At the same time as this may not continually speed up the hair increase method, slumbering on a silk pillowcase generates tons less friction and offers hair a softer surface to relax on.

Use Keratin-based products to fill in Breakage

It's proper that keratin-primarily based completely products can combat dryness and make the hair appear shinier; but, it may also enhance the hair and save your future breakage from occurring.

The protein, which is shielding in nature, douses hair in critical oils and vitamins it desires to thrive, creating extraordinary surroundings for wholesome strands to grow.

Chapter 2:

Unique ingredients that works effectively on Hair mask

Hair masks run the gamut in terms of elements that could provide your hair a few TLC. The components that may go exquisite for you could depend on your hair kind and the situation of your hair and scalp.

Right here are a number of the maximum well-known additives to search for in a store-supplied mask or to check with whilst making your very own:

Bananas: if you want to reduce frizz, bananas are an outstanding element to consist of in a hair mask. The silica in bananas also can assist make your hair softer and shinier. In step with 2011 take a look at relied on deliver, bananas additionally have antimicrobial homes. This may help reduce dryness and dandruff.

Eggs: The vitamins in egg yolks, which include nutrients A and E, biotin, and foliate, may also help sell hair increase, at the same time as the protein in egg whites may additionally assist beef up your hair.

Avocado oil: The minerals in avocado oil, which consist of folic acid, iron, and magnesium, might also assist seal the hair cuticle. This can assist make your hair extra immune to harm and breakage.

Honey: Honey is considered humectants, which means that it is able to help your hair pull in and preserve more moisture. It is able to additionally stimulate the boom of pores and skin cells trusted supply, which may additionally assist sell stronger hair follicles.

Coconut oil: this may assist reduce dryness and frizz. Research from 2015Trusted sources has moreover shown that coconut oil can lessen protein loss whilst used on the hair.

Olive oil: need extreme moisture? Olive oil includes squalene, which's produced definitely with the resource of the body, but, declines as we age. Squalene is essential for moisturized hair and pores and skin.

Aloe-Vera: in case you want to calm and soothe your scalp, don't forget a hair mask with aloe Vera, which has anti-inflammatory residences. It is usually nutrients C, E, and B-12, folic acid, and choline, which may assist make it more potent and nourish your hair.

Chapter 3:

Recipes for Hair mask

Making your very own hair masks is quite smooth and maybe a laugh, too. If you haven't attempted a hair mask earlier, you could want to check with a few one-of-a-kind recipes and components until you find the simplest one that's excellently suitable on your hair.

You'll are aware of it's a great fit in case your hair feels smooth and moisturized without looking or feeling greasy or limp.

To get commenced, you may want to know the form of simple but effective DIY hair mask recipes. You can grow the quantity of the materials, relying on the duration of your hair.

For frizzy or damaged hair

Additives:

1 tbsp. natural uncooked honey

1 tbsp. herbal coconut oil

Instructions:

Warmth the honey and coconut oil together in a saucepan

Stir till combined.

Permit the combination to chill, after which applies it to your hair.

Permit it to take a seat for forty mins, then shampoo and condition as normal.

For dry hair or dandruff

Factors:

1 ripe avocado

2 tbsp. of aloe Vera gel

1 tsp. of coconut oil

Commands:

Combo the 3 materials collectively, then apply to wet or dry hair from root to tip.

Allow it to take a seat for a half-hour, after which rinse with lukewarm water.

For excellent, thinning hair

Substances:

2 egg whites

2 tbsp. coconut oil

Instructions:

Mix egg together thoroughly with oil

Observe from root to tip to damp hair, and permit it to take a seat for 20 mins.

Shampoo with cold water

This is especially crucial for masks that encompass egg, as heat water can motive the egg to cook inside the hair.

Chapter 4:

Ways you should apply hair mask

Most hair mask artwork quality whilst implemented to clean, towel-dried hair that's though damp

But, in case you're the use of a hair mask made typically of oil, like coconut or olive oil, it may be satisfactory to use the masks to dry hair. Because of the truth oil can repel water; some hair care experts consider that dry hair is able to absorb the oil better than wet hair.

As quickly because the hair masks are geared up to apply, comply with these steps:

To protect your clothing, drape a vintage towel over your shoulders or put on a vintage T-shirt.

If your hair is lengthy or thick, it is able to help to divide it into sections with hair clips.

You may practice the mask in conjunction with your hands, or you can use a small paintbrush to dab the hair masks mixture onto your hair.

If your hair is dry, start the hair masks software program

close to your scalp and artwork in the direction of the ends. Once the mask was worked into the ends of your hair, you could bypass decrease again and lightly observe on your scalp.

In case you're especially making use of the masks to deal with dandruff, you'll need to begin at your scalp.

If your hair is oily, start the hair mask utility at mid-shaft and artwork in the direction of the ends.

While you're completed utilizing the masks, run a huge-teeth comb thru your hair to assist ensure the mask are evenly spread.

Cover your hair with a tub cap or plastic wrap. Then wrap a towel spherical to your head. This helps shield the masks from dripping, however, it also facilitates add some warmth, which could assist the elements to absorb into your hair.

Go away the masks on for at least 20 to half of-hour. Counting on the elements, some masks can be left on for hours or even in a single day.

Rinse very well with lukewarm or cool water. Avoid heat water. Cooler water can assist seal the hair cuticle and help your hair keep greater moisture.

After rinsing out the masks — it is able to take or greater rinses to get it absolutely out — you can upload merchandise and air-dry or warm temperature-fashion your hair as standard.

For dry, frizzy, or damaged hair, you may have a look at a hair ask once consistent with the week. If your hair has a tendency to be oilier, strive the use one each couple of weeks.

Chapter 5:

The kind of natural shampoo recipe you should avoid

DIY shampoo recipes are so popular proper now! but, the choice for easy, natural recipes made from additives you'll discover in your kitchen, has caused a ton of recipes being shared online that definitely gained paintings, (and can even do harm to your hair).

This text will provide an explanation for what's incorrect with the most well-known types of DIY shampoo recipe and we'll percent what powerful recipe dreams rather.

DIY hair care recipes are generally based definitely around the subsequent ingredients:

Castile soap

Coconut milk

Cold system cleansing soap bars

Baking soda

No longer handiest do those recipes now not effectively

cleanse and shield the hair, (extra on that during a minute), there are exceptional risks related to the usage of them too. for example, the good-sized majority of DIY recipes aren't preserved or stored correctly, which can cause microorganisms, yeast, and mold to proliferate in them – probably main to pores and skin and eye infections, thrush, toxic surprise, and atopic dermatitis.

Before we pass any further, allows observing what an effective shampoo need to do.

Cleanse the hair: Shampoo allows the elimination of dirt and soil from the hair and scalp. Sebum, dust, and styling merchandise building up on hair through the years and shampoo are wanted to remove them, without being too harsh and casting off beneficial lipids on the hair.

If the tiles are well-closed or laid down, they shield the underneath floor. A first-rate shampoo will make sure that cells of the cuticle are laid flat, for that reason shielding the below layers from harm.

Stability pH of hair: Hair needs a barely acidic pH in order for the cuticle to be closed down, and to decrease the static power which motives tangles and damage to the hair.

1) Castile soap

A huge quantity of DIY Shampoo recipes uses Castile cleaning soap as their essential aspect, regularly blended with aloe Vera, carrier oils, and/or vital oils. We apprehend why humans assume they might use it – it foams, (a chunk), it cleanses the scalp, it's smooth to get hold of, and it's manifestly derived. It's a remarkable, simple purifier for pores and skin. But what about hair

Is Castile cleansing cleaning soap a suitable shampoo? Does it cleanse the hair, close the cuticle, and stabilize the pH?

Castile soap will sincerely cleanse the hair, so this undertaking is looked after. But it received does the alternative responsibilities – the pH of Castile cleaning soap can be very immoderate (or alkaline – the alternative of acidic), round nine -10, that is completely improper for hair. Even as hair is handled with an alkaline product, it'll leave the cuticle cells open and vulnerable to harm. Hair with an imbalanced pH also can be lots more liable to breaking and tangling.

Global satisfactory homemade Shampoo (that's best to your hair kind)

Elements:

About ¾ cup liquid Castile cleaning soap

¼ cup aloe vera.

1 tsp jojoba oil

½ – 1 tsp sweet almond oil (non-compulsory for dry hair)

50-60 drops of essential oils of your choice (nice in your hair type)

What's incorrect with this recipe?

Similarly to the maximum crucial problem with Castile cleaning soap, as described above, this shampoo has some different troubles to the phrase:

It does not include a preservative – if this combination is left at room temperature for numerous days, its miles very likely to show microbial growth in it – yikes!

It mixes oil and water – factors that may be incompatible without an emulsifier or solubilizer.

The recipe suggests that including crucial oils will make it "ideal on your hair kind". At the same time as changing the vital oils can exchange the residences of a product piece, to honestly adjust the product to your hair kind; tons more than changing important oils are wished. You need to don't forget which cleansing sellers to apply and the amount wanted, and consider which special nurturing components are appropriate for that hair kind. Additionally, which type of shampoo ought to be formulated within the first vicinity?

It uses inconsistent and misguided measurements. Drops, cups, teaspoons, and such aren't accurate measurements for relaxed and powerful cosmetic formulations.

Shampoo cleaning soap bars

Many DIY recipes are for 'stable shampoo bars, which at the closer inspection are honestly bloodless process cleansing cleaning soap bars. 'Soaping' is, in reality, a popular (and addictive!) hobby for lots. Self-made cold technique soap can be high-quality for your pores and skin. But, is it any properly for hair?

Cleansing soap bars are very much like liquid Castile cleaning soap; however, they have got a sturdy shape. The chemistry at the back of that merchandise is identical and that they each have a pH this is manner too excessive for the hair. soap bars will ease the hair correctly, but in view that they gained close to the cuticle down or balance the pH of the hair, it's going to leave the hair dry, tangled, and at risk of further harm.

Here's an instance of a web self-made stable shampoo bar recipe:

Additives:

10 oz. coconut oil

10 ounces tallow (or palm oil)

10 oz. olive oil

6 oz... Castor oil

5 ozlye

12 ounces distilled water

1.5 ounces of crucial oils introduced at hint

This is truly a nice recipe for cold gadget cleansing cleaning soap with the intention to make an incredible cleansing cleaning soap bar for use on palms and frame, however not at the hair!

4) Baking soda

Every other well-known category of DIY shampoo uses baking soda as an essential aspect element. It's smooth to get maintain of, (you likely already have some), and it's less high-priced. However is baking soda a suitable shampoo? Does it cleanse the hair, near the cuticle, balance the pH?

Baking soda can act as a degreaser, so it will remove a number of the oils from the hair; however, it gained does it very gently. An answer of baking soda in water has a very immoderate pH, (approximately 95), which's too high for the hair and may irritate your scalp. It going to now not near the cuticle, and will in the end departs your hair brittle and prone to breakage.

We discovered those commands for a baking soda shampoo:

"Begin with the useful resource of blending 1 element baking soda with 3 components water. i have shoulder duration hair and blend approximately 2 to a few tablespoons of baking soda with 3 times that amount of water in a small squeeze bottle. You may regulate this by way of counting on your hair period. Exercise the baking soda and water mixture to dry or moist hair with the resource of beginning on the roots and operating to the ends. Allow it sit down for 1 – three mins, and then rinse with warm water."

As said above, this method might also offer some degreasing, but, may even motive damage to the hair. So it is not a first-rate opportunity for herbal shampoo.

Chapter 6

The after effect of using Apple cider vinegar for hair growth

Apple cider vinegar (ACV) is a famous condiment and health food. It's crafted from apples using a fermentation way enriching it with stay cultures, minerals, and acids.

ACV has many packages as a home cure. This type is a hair wash to enhance scalp health, make more potent hair, and enhance shine.

Even as hailed as a domestic "panacea" or "remedy-all" for health issues despite being underneath-researched, the blessings and technological know-how spherical ACV does deliver as regards hair care.

For those handling hair issues at the side of itchy scalp or hair breakage, apple cider vinegar might be a splendid herbal treatment to discover.

How do I take ACV for hair care?

An ACV wash can be made very without a doubt.

Rinse it out.

Coconuts and Kettle bells suggest blending some drops of vital oil into the mixture if the acidic smell is just too effective for you. The scent must additionally leave rapid after rinsing.

Strive to incorporate the rinse into your hair care routine a couple of instances per week. Also, sense loose to boom the quantity of ACV you use in every wash or rinse. Generally, preserving it around five tablespoons or less is normally advocated.

What to pay attention to:

Using apple cider vinegar is all approximately bringing hair again into stability. In case your hair or scalp issues worsen as an alternative, prevent the usage of ACV. Or, strive to lessen the quantity you positioned right into a rinse, or the frequency you use it.

Apple cider vinegar consists of acetic acids recognized to be caustic. This means they will get worse or burn the pores and pores and skin.

Always dilute ACV with water earlier than making use of it at once to the skin. If your rinses are too sturdy, attempt to dilute it greater — even though if the infection takes place, it almost always clears up internally a couple of days

Also, avoid contact with eyes. If contact happens, rapidly wash out with water.

<u>THE END</u>

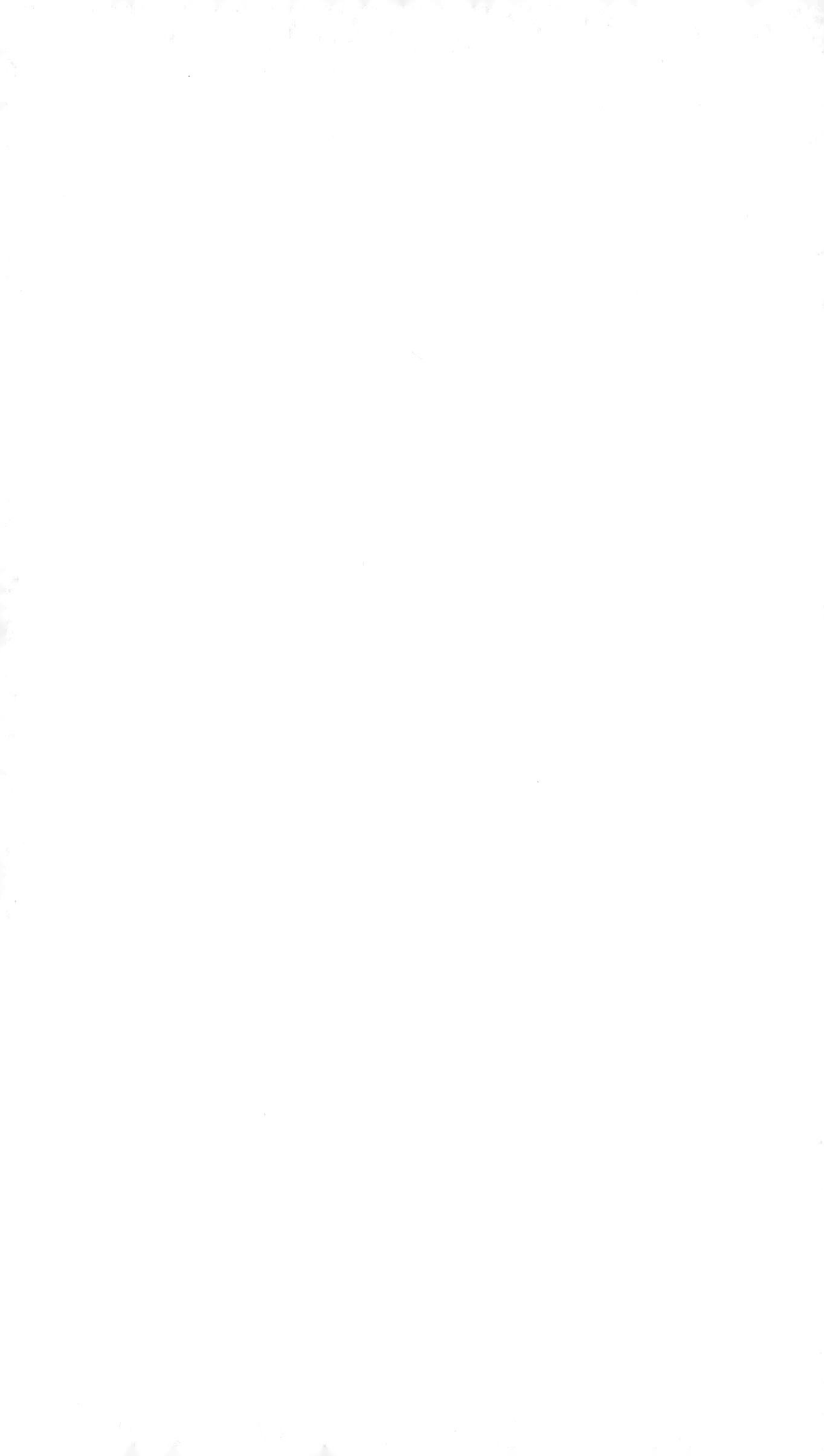